Acknowledgn

D1633944

We would like to thank those who have been helpful to us in the completion of this project.

- Our thanks to Andrew Allen, Mary Jo Adams, and the Elsevier editorial team for their guidance and providing the necessary resources to complete this project.
- Our thanks to Dr. Greg Lachar, Andrew Baird, Andrea Lowrey, Paul Honeywell, and Jay Wood for providing many of the 12-lead ECGs used in this pocket reference.

Tim Phalen
Barb Aehlert

Acknowledgments

We would like to thank those who have been helpful to us in the completion of this project.

Our thanks to Andrew Allen, Steve Jo Amirav, and the Elsevier editorial team for their guidance and providing the necessary resources to complete this project.

Our thanks to Dr. Gary Keller, Andrew Boyd, Andrew Carey, Paul Stockwell, and Jay Wood for providing many of the 12-Lead ECG used in this pocket reference.

Tim Phalen
Paris Achbet

Contents

Contents

Suspecting STEMI

aVR   V1

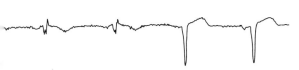

IDENTIFICATION

The J-point

As its name implies, recognition of an ST-segment elevation myocardial infarction (STEMI) requires analysis of the ST segment. The earliest portion of the ST segment is called the ST-junction or J-point. The J-point is the point where the QRS ends and the ST begins. It is at the J-point where ST analysis is performed (Figure 1-1).

One way to locate the J-point is described here. Select a representative P-QRS-T sequence. Do not select an ectopic beat. The P-QRS-T sequence selected should have with a steady baseline preceding and following it. Follow the QRS complex to its end. The point where the QRS ends and changes direction is the J-point. Figure 1-2 highlights the J-point in a variety of QRS morphologies.

ST-segment elevation provides the strongest ECG evidence for the early recognition of myocardial infarction (MI). Table 1-1 reflects current criteria for ST-segment displacement.

STEMI Recognition – Goal #1:
When you claim ST elevation is present, it is. When you claim ST elevation is not present, it is not.

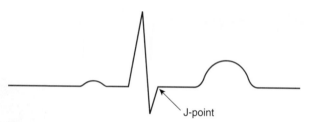

Figure 1-1   The point where the QRS complex and the ST-segment meet is called the *ST-junction* or *J-point.*

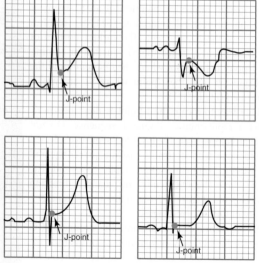

Figure 1-2   Examples of QRS complexes with the J-point identified.

Table **1-1**	ST-Segment Displacement[1]		
Patient	ECG Lead	Threshold Value for Abnormal J-point Elevation	Threshold Value for Abnormal J-point Depression
Male, 40 years and older	V_2 and V_3 All other leads	2 mm 1 mm	0.5 mm 1 mm
Male, less than 40 years old	V_2 and V_3 All other leads	2.5 mm 1 mm	0.5 mm 1 mm
Female	V_2 and V_3 All other leads	1.5 mm More than 1 mm	0.5 mm 1 mm
Male, 30 years and older	V_3R and V_4R	0.5 mm	1 mm
Male, less than 30 years old	V_3R and V_4R	1 mm	1 mm
Female	V_3R and V_4R	0.5 mm	1 mm
Male and female	V_7 through V_9	0.5 mm	1 mm

The presence of ST-segment elevation is sometimes obvious. At other times it may seem that the ST segment is elevated when in fact it is not—at least not in a way that meets the current criteria in the STEMI guidelines. Look at Figure 1-3. Many of these complexes may at first glance appear to meet the ST-segment elevation criteria. In fact, none of them do.

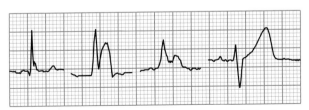

Figure 1-3 Examples of complexes that appear to meet ST elevation criteria but do not.

Once the J-point has been correctly identified, the next task is to determine if it is elevated. To do this, you must compare the J-point to the baseline and determine if elevation is present. Several factors can affect the position of portions of the baseline. For example, if the PR segment is depressed, it may give the appearance or illusion of ST elevation when in fact ST elevation is not present (Figure 1-4). Therefore when assessing for ST elevation, compare the J-point to the TP segment.

On the ECG grid, the smallest box is 1 millimeter (mm) in size. Once the J-point has been located and compared to the TP segment, determine if the J-point is displaced by 1 mm or more above the level of the TP segment (Figure 1-5). Look at the 12-lead ECG in Figure 1-6 and determine which leads display J-point elevation of 1 mm or more.

The current criteria for the STEMI Guidelines call for ST elevation of 1 mm or more in two anatomically contiguous leads. *Contiguous* means "neighboring" or "adjoining." To meet the STEMI criteria, one must find ST elevation in two ECG leads that "view" neighboring or adjoining tissue in the heart itself.

Unfortunately, in the standard 12-lead ECG, the leads are not printed in relation to the heart's anatomy. To be clear, what matters is which part of the heart each lead "sees" and not the lead's location on the 12-lead printout. Leads can be next to each other in the ECG printout but not "look" at contiguous tissue in

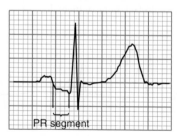

Figure 1-4   If the PR segment is depressed, it may give the appearance or illusion of ST elevation when in fact ST elevation is not present.

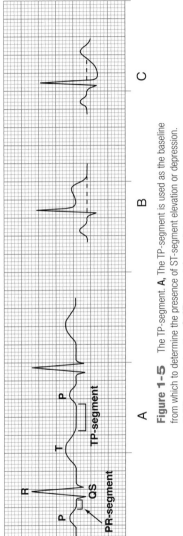

Figure 1-5 The TP-segment. **A,** The TP-segment is used as the baseline from which to determine the presence of ST-segment elevation or depression. **B,** ST-segment elevation. **C,** ST-segment depression.

Figure 1-6 Which leads show ST elevation of 1 millimeter or more?

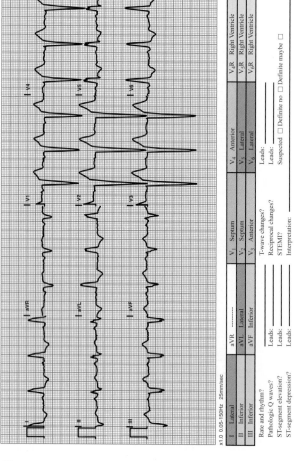

x1.0 0.05-150Hz 25mm/sec

I	Lateral	aVR	----------	V₁	Septum	V₄	Anterior	V₄R	Right Ventricle
II	Inferior	aVL	Lateral	V₂	Septum	V₅	Lateral	V₅R	Right Ventricle
III	Inferior	aVF	Inferior	V₃	Anterior	V₆	Lateral	V₆R	Right Ventricle

Rate and rhythm: _____
Pathologic Q waves? _____
ST-segment elevation? _____
ST-segment depression? _____

T-wave changes? _____
Reciprocal changes? _____
STEMI? _____
Interpretation: _____

Leads: _____
Leads: _____
Suspected ☐ Definite no ☐ Definite maybe ☐

the heart. Therefore in order to suspect STEMI, we need to know which part of the heart each lead "sees."

Lead Views

Electrodes are not "leads," and neither are the cables or wires. Each electrode picks up a signal from the heart. Leads are specific combinations of those signals. A lead is a combination of a ground or reference, one positive signal, and one, two, or three negative signals. Figure 1-7 shows how the electrodes are used as the positive signal for each lead. One electrode can be used as the positive signal for multiple leads.

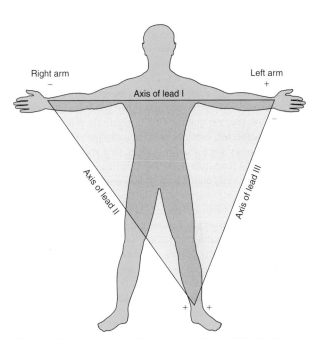

Figure 1-7   In a standard 12-lead electrocardiogram (ECG), all 12 leads are obtained from 10 electrodes positioned as shown here.

While leads are not really cameras or eyes, it can be useful to think of them as such when considering which anatomic region is associated with each lead. Each lead has one and only one positive electrode and that positive electrode can be thought of as a camera or an eye. Where that positive electrode is placed on the body determines which part of the heart it will "see" (Figure 1-8, Table 1-2).

The color overlay provided with the full text allows you to place the overlay on top of an ECG. The colors help to determine which part of the heart each leads "sees" (Figure 1-9).

Of the 12 standard ECG leads, lead aVR is not used in the same way for STEMI recognition. From its position on the right arm, lead aVR sees the chamber or cavity of the left ventricle. All of the other leads are influenced by a specific portion the outer tissue of the left ventricle, which is influenced by a specific portion of the epicardium. Because aVR is influenced by endocardium, we do not use it in the same way for STEMI recognition and localization.

One of the uses for aVR is to identify potential misplaced limb lead cables. The QRS complex in aVR is expected to be negative—that is, primarily below the baseline. When you look at the tracing in lead aVR, confirm that the QRS is negatively deflected. If it is negatively deflected, continue with your interpretation. However, if the QRS in aVR is primarily upright, stop your interpretation and check the four limb lead cables and confirm that they are positioned correctly on the body. If they are positioned correctly, continue with your interpretation. If they are not positioned correctly, reposition them and run a new ECG.

When ST elevation (J-point elevation) is noted in two leads that are anatomically contiguous, STEMI can be suspected as a possibility. The most common way of assessing if two leads are contiguous is if they are two leads of the same anatomic group. For example, if any two of the inferior leads show ST elevation, then STEMI can be suspected (the actual likelihood that ST elevation is from STEMI is discussed in Chapter 2).

Leads are considered anatomically contiguous if they are assigned to the same anatomic group—for example, ST elevation

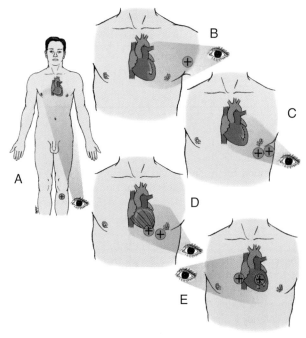

Figure 1-8 **A,** Leads II, III, and aVF each has a positive electrode posi-tioned on the left leg. From the perspective of the left leg, each of them "sees" the inferior wall of the left ventricle. **B,** From their vantage point on the left arm, leads I and aVL "look" in at the lateral wall of the left ventricle. **C,** Leads V$_5$ and V$_6$ also "view" the lateral wall because they are positioned on the axillary area of the left chest. **D,** Leads V$_3$ and V$_4$ are positioned in the area of the anterior chest. From this perspective, these leads "see" the anterior wall of the left ventricle. **E,** The septal wall is "seen" by leads V$_1$ and V$_2$, which are positioned next to the sternum.

in two inferior leads, two anterior leads, etc. This is the most common means by which leads are identified as contiguous. Occasionally, however, there is an exception. This exception only applies to the chest leads (leads V$_1$–V$_6$). Here is the excep-tion: If ST elevation is noted in two numerically consecutive

Table **1-2** What Each Lead "Sees"	
Leads	Heart Surface Viewed
II, III, aVF	Inferior
V_1, V_2	Septal
V_3, V_4	Anterior
I, aVL, V_5, V_6	Lateral

chest leads, suspect STEMI. That is, each chest lead is contiguous with its neighbor. For example, suppose you identified ST elevation in V_2 and V_3 but nowhere else. Lead V_2 views the septal wall and lead V_3 sees the anterior wall. At first glance, it may appear that ST elevation is not present in two anatomically contiguous leads. Upon further reflection, you remember that if ST elevation is present in two *numerically* contiguous chest leads, they are also contiguous. This makes sense if you consider that the "cameras" or "eyes" are located right next to each other on the patient's chest. Of course they will see contiguous tissue in the heart. So, leads are considered anatomically contiguous if they are of the same group (two inferior leads, two anterior leads, etc,) or if they are numerically consecutive chest leads (V_1 is contiguous with V_2, V_2 is contiguous with both V_1 and V_3, etc.).

Putting these concepts together, we can now *suspect* STEMI. Before examining the 12-lead for ECG evidence of possible STEMI, it is appropriate to have first determined rate and rhythm. Once rate and rhythm have been determined (often before the 12-lead was obtained), systematically examine each lead checking for ST-segment elevation. Remember to use the J-point and the TP segment in each lead when making this determination. You can skip aVR for the moment.

When you have examined all of the leads, ask yourself, "Did I find ST-segment elevation in two anatomically contiguous leads?" If the answer is yes, then you may *suspect* STEMI and even be able to localize that suspected STEMI. Localizing refers to determining which coronary artery (and corresponding tissue) is most likely affected.

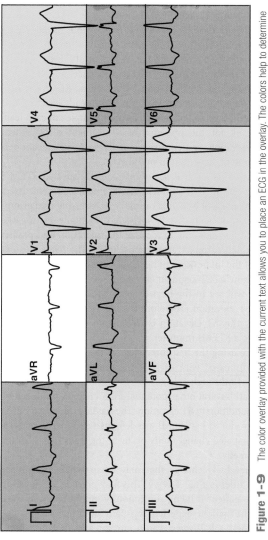

Figure 1-9 The color overlay provided with the current text allows you to place an ECG in the overlay. The colors help to determine which part of the heart each lead "sees."

Here are the first three steps of a five-step approach to use when analyzing a 12-lead ECG.

Step 1. *Identify the rate and underlying rhythm.* Determining rate and rhythm is the first priority when interpreting the ECG. Remember, the treatment of life-threatening dysrhythmias initially takes precedence over the acquisition and interpretation of the 12-lead ECG.

Step 2. *Analyze waveforms.* Examine each lead, selecting one good representative waveform or complex in each lead. Look for the presence of ST-segment displacement (elevation or depression). If ST-segment elevation is present, express it in millimeters.

Step 3. *Examine for evidence of infarction.* Suspected STEMI? Location? If ST-segment displacement is present, assess the areas of ischemia or injury by assessing lead groupings. If acute MI is suspected, mentally picture the cardiac anatomy to localize the infarction and predict which coronary artery is occluded. The relative extent of the infarction can be gauged by the number of leads showing ST-segment elevation.

As we will see in the next chapter, STEMI is not the only cause of ST elevation. Therefore the next step is to determine how likely this ST elevation is to be from genuine STEMI as opposed to a STEMI imposter.

Practice using the first three steps of the five-step approach we have discussed with each of the practice ECGs provided (Figures 1-10 through 1-14).

There are several other potential ECG changes produced by STEMI in addition to ST elevation. The classic evolutionary ECG changes produced by STEMI are demonstrated in Figure 1-15. These anticipated changes only occur in the leads that "see" the STEMI directly.

The first ECG change that may occur when a coronary artery occludes is a tall T wave. This may precede ST elevation and, if the patient is being continuously monitored, may even precede the patient experiencing pain or other complaints. Because these tall T waves can occur so early, they are sometimes referred to as hyperacute T waves. A T wave is considered

text continues on page 19

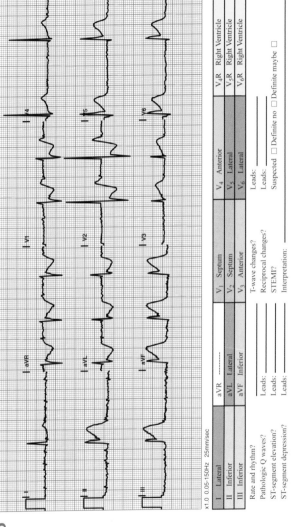

x1.0 0.05-150Hz 25mm/sec

I Lateral	aVR --------	V₁ Septum	V₄ Anterior	V₄R Right Ventricle
II Inferior	aVL Lateral	V₂ Septum	V₅ Lateral	V₅R Right Ventricle
III Inferior	aVF Inferior	V₃ Anterior	V₆ Lateral	V₆R Right Ventricle

Rate and rhythm? _____

Pathologic Q waves? Leads: _____

ST-segment elevation? Leads: _____

ST-segment depression? Leads: _____

T-wave changes? Leads: _____

Reciprocal changes? Leads: _____

STEMI? Suspected ☐ Definite no ☐ Definite maybe ☐

Interpretation: _____

Figure 1-10

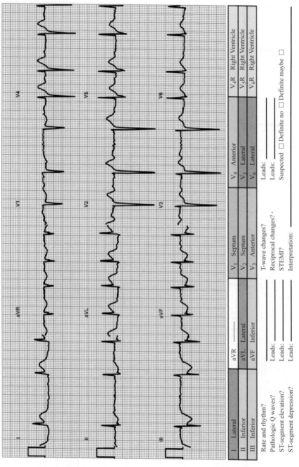

I Lateral	aVR	V₁ Septum	V₄ Anterior	V₄R Right Ventricle
II Inferior	aVL Lateral	V₂ Septum	V₅ Lateral	V₅R Right Ventricle
III Inferior	aVF Inferior	V₃ Anterior	V₆ Lateral	V₆R Right Ventricle

Rate and rhythm? _____   T-wave changes? _____   Leads: _____

Pathologic Q waves? Leads: _____   Reciprocal changes? · Leads: _____   Leads: _____

ST-segment elevation? Leads: _____   STEMI? _____   Suspected ☐ Definite no ☐ Definite maybe ☐

ST-segment depression? Leads: _____   Interpretation: _____

Figure 1–11

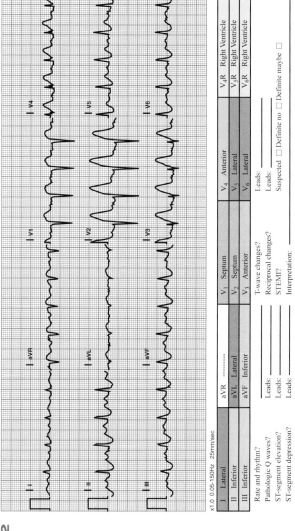

Figure 1-12

x1.0 0.05-150Hz 25mm/sec

I	Lateral	aVR	....	V₁	Septum	V₄	Anterior	V₄R	Right Ventricle
II	Inferior	aVL	Lateral	V₂	Septum	V₅	Lateral	V₅R	Right Ventricle
III	Inferior	aVF	Inferior	V₃	Anterior	V₆	Lateral	V₆R	Right Ventricle

Rate and rhythm: _____

Pathologic Q waves?   Leads: _____   T-wave changes? _____   Leads: _____
ST-segment elevation?   Leads: _____   Reciprocal changes? _____   Leads: _____
ST-segment depression?   Leads: _____   STEMI? _____

Interpretation: _____

Suspected ☐ Definite no ☐ Definite maybe ☐

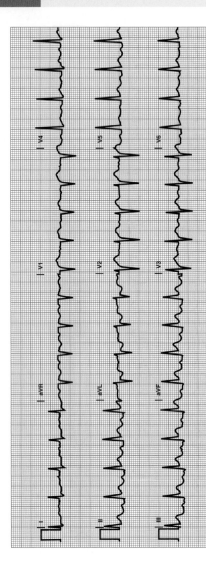

x1.0 0.05-150Hz 25mm/sec

I Lateral	aVR	V₁ Septum	V₄ Anterior	V₄R Right Ventricle
II Inferior	aVL Lateral	V₂ Septum	V₅ Lateral	V₅R Right Ventricle
III Inferior	aVF Inferior	V₃ Anterior	V₆ Lateral	V₆R Right Ventricle

Rate and rhythm? _____

Pathologic Q waves? Leads: _____

ST-segment elevation? Leads: _____

ST-segment depression? Leads: _____

T-wave changes? _____

Reciprocal changes? _____

STEMI? _____

Interpretation: _____

Leads: _____

Leads: _____

Suspected ☐ Definite no ☐ Definite maybe ☐

Figure 1-13

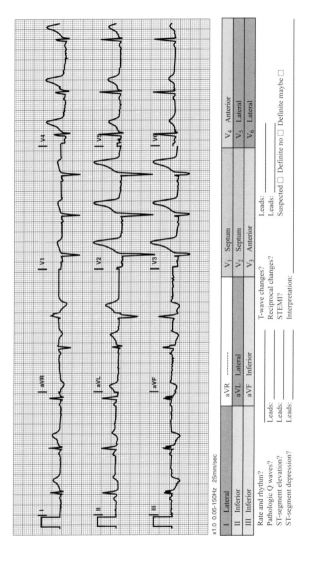

x1.0 0.05-150Hz 25mm/sec

I Lateral	aVR -------	V₁ Septum	V₄ Anterior
II Inferior	aVL Lateral	V₂ Septum	V₅ Lateral
III Inferior	aVF Inferior	V₃ Anterior	V₆ Lateral

Rate and rhythm? _____

Pathologic Q waves? Leads: ____

ST-segment elevation? Leads: ____

ST-segment depression? Leads: ____

T-wave changes? Leads: ____

Reciprocal changes? Leads: ____

STEMI? Suspected ☐ Definite no ☐ Definite maybe ☐

Interpretation: _____

Figure
1-14

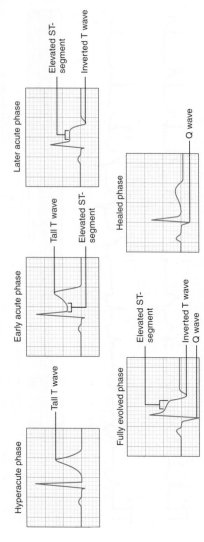

Figure 1-15 The evolving pattern of ST-elevation myocardial infarction on the ECG.

tall if it is more than 5 mm (one big box) in the limb leads (I, II, III aVL, and aVF) and more than 10 mm in the chest leads (V_1–V_6).

Over time, ST-segment elevation may develop, indicating myocardial injury in progress. ST elevation may occur within the first hour or first few hours of infarction. We have already discussed how to recognize ST elevation. In the later acute phase of the infarction, you may see the presence of T-wave inversion, suggesting the presence of ischemia. In fact, T-wave inversion may precede the development of ST-segment elevation, or they may occur at the same time.

If the tissue hypoxia that produced the tissue injury persists, tissue death may result. The ECG evidence associated with dead myocardial tissue is an abnormal (pathologic) Q wave. The components of a normal QRS complex are identified in Figure 1-16. Note that a Q wave is a negative deflection preceding the R wave. In some leads, Q waves may be an expected part of a normal ECG. In other cases, however, a Q wave may be the result of pathology, such as myocardial tissue death (Figure 1-17).

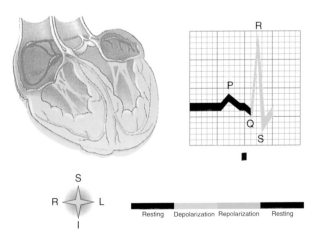

Figure 1-16   The QRS complex represents ventricular depolarization.

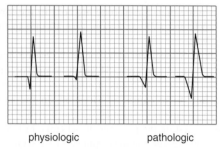

physiologic   pathologic

Figure 1-17   Physiologic and pathologic Q waves.

Pathologic Q waves tend to be wider and/or deeper than physiologic Q waves. When a Q wave is noted, measure the width of the Q wave itself (not the entire QRS complex). If the width is 0.04 second or more, suspect the Q wave to be pathologic, and possibly the ECG evidence of dead myocardial tissue.

When both ST elevation and a pathologic Q wave are noted on a 12-lead ECG, the STEMI may still be acute, which means that it may still be ongoing. There may very well be some jeopardized myocardium that can still be saved. Therefore the appearance of a pathologic Q wave does not mean the STEMI is over and has run its course. When ST elevation is present, with or without a pathologic Q wave, consider it to be acute until proved otherwise.

When the entire process of an MI has completed, the ST segment is expected to return to the baseline. A pathologic Q wave, however, may remain as evidence of a previous MI. From this point on the age of the infarction cannot be estimated from the ECG. It is thus considered to be *age undetermined*. It could be a day old or a decade old.

It is important to note that while the pattern demonstrated in Figure 1-15 is the "classic" evolutionary ECG pattern of STEMI, many STEMI patients will vary at least somewhat from this pattern. Learn the evolutionary pattern of STEMI, use it as a reference, and compare findings to that reference, but remember that *a normal ECG does not rule out myocardial infarction!*

Until now all of our discussion has been about the ECG changes occurring in the leads "looking" directly at the STEMI. But remember—you have electrodes all over the patient and some of them are going to see the STEMI from the opposite perspective. When you see something backward, you often see things from a different perspective. That is what reciprocal changes are (Figure 1-18). For example, when a positive electrode sees the STEMI head on, it may produce ST elevation. If a different lead saw the same STEMI from the opposite perspective, then it might demonstrate an opposite set of changes, or ST depression. If a lead

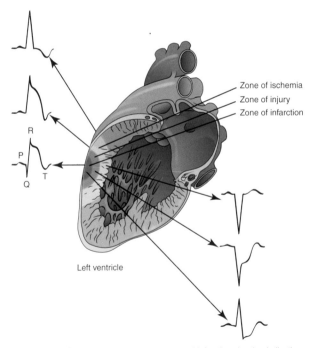

Zone of ischemia
Zone of injury
Zone of infarction

Left ventricle

Figure 1-18 Zones of ischemia, injury, and infarction showing indicative ECG changes and reciprocal changes corresponding to each zone.

sees a STEMI head on and a tall T wave is noted, then the leads seeing the event backward will show an inverted T wave. Which leads oppose which? Table 1-3 shows where to look for reciprocal changes.

It is important to note that not all STEMIs produce reciprocal changes. Some do, some do not. It is not necessary to see reciprocal changes to suspect STEMI. However, if clear and obvious reciprocal changes are present, that is an important ECG change to note. Look at the ECGs in Figures 1-19 through 1-21 and decide if reciprocal changes are present.

At this point we can expand our systematic approach a bit further. When you examine each lead of the 12-lead ECG, look for the following: pathologic Q waves, ST elevation, ST depression, tall T waves, and inverted T waves. This rounds out the list of classic ECG changes produced by STEMI. In the next chapter, we will add the last two steps in our five-step approach to 12-lead analysis.

Table 1-3 Localization of a Myocardial Infarction

Location of MI	Indicative Changes (Leads facing affected area)	Reciprocal Changes (Leads opposite affected area)	Affected (Culprit) Coronary Artery
Anterior	V_3, V_4	V_7, V_8, V_9	Left coronary artery • LAD—diagonal branch
Anteroseptal	V_1, V_2, V_3, V_4	V_7, V_8, V_9	Left coronary artery • LAD—diagonal branch • LAD—septal branch
Anterolateral	I, aVL, V_3, V_4, V_5, V_6	II, III, aVF, V_7, V_8, V_9	Left coronary artery • LAD—diagonal branch and/or • Circumflex branch
Inferior	II, III, aVF	I, aVL	Right coronary artery (most common) — posterior descending branch or Left coronary artery—circumflex branch
Lateral	I, aVL, V_5, V_6	II, III, aVF	Left coronary artery • LAD—diagonal branch and/or • Circumflex branch Right coronary artery
Septum	V_1, V_2	V_7, V_8, V_9	Left coronary artery • LAD—septal branch
Posterior	V_7, V_8, V_9	V_1, V_2, V_3	Right coronary or circumflex artery
Right ventricle	V_1R–V_6R	I, aVL	Right coronary artery • Proximal branches

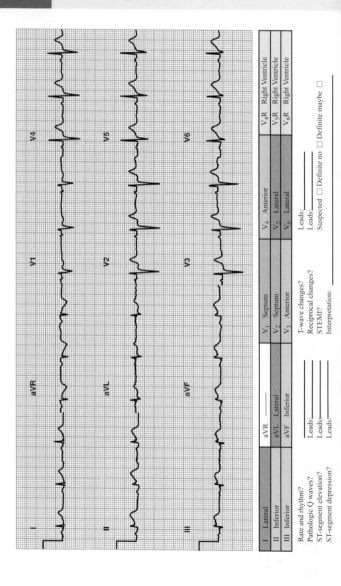

I	Lateral	aVR	-------	V₁	Septum	V₄	Anterior	V₄R	Right Ventricle
II	Inferior	aVL	Lateral	V₂	Septum	V₅	Lateral	V₅R	Right Ventricle
III	Inferior	aVF	Inferior	V₃	Anterior	V₆	Lateral	V₆R	Right Ventricle

Rate and rhythm? _____
Pathologic Q waves?   Leads: _____
ST-segment elevation?   Leads: _____
ST-segment depression?   Leads: _____

T-wave changes? _____
Reciprocal changes? _____
STEMI? _____
Interpretation: _____

Leads: _____
Leads: _____
Suspected ☐ Definite no ☐ Definite maybe ☐

Figure
1-19

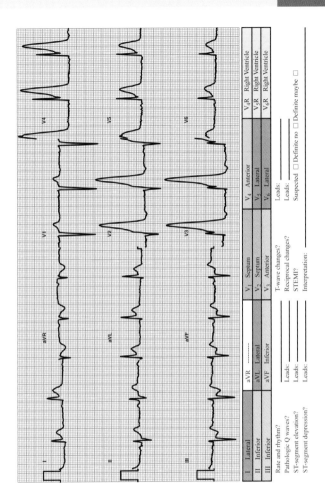

I	Lateral	aVR	--------	V₁	Septum	V₄	Anterior	V₄R	Right Ventricle
II	Inferior	aVL	Lateral	V₂	Septum	V₅	Lateral	V₅R	Right Ventricle
III	Inferior	aVF	Inferior	V₃	Anterior	V₆	Lateral	V₆R	Right Ventricle

Rate and rhythm? _____
Pathologic Q waves? _____ Leads: _____
ST-segment elevation? _____ Leads: _____
ST-segment depression? _____ Leads: _____

T-wave changes? _____
Reciprocal changes? _____ Leads: _____
STEMI? _____ Leads: _____
Interpretation: _____

Suspected □ Definite no □ Definite maybe □

Figure 1-20

Figure 1-21

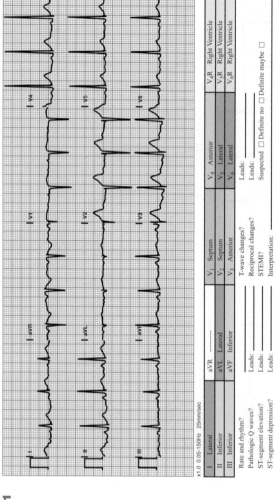

x1.0 0.05-150Hz 25mm/sec

I	Lateral	aVR	---------	V₁	Septum	V₄	Anterior	V₄R	Right Ventricle
II	Inferior	aVL	Lateral	V₂	Septum	V₅	Lateral	V₅R	Right Ventricle
III	Inferior	aVF	Inferior	V₃	Anterior	V₆	Lateral	V₆R	Right Ventricle

Rate and rhythm? _____

Pathologic Q waves? Leads: _____

ST-segment elevation? Leads: _____

ST-segment depression? Leads: _____

T-wave changes? Leads: _____

Reciprocal changes? Leads: _____

STEMI? _____

Interpretation: _____

Suspected ☐ Definite no ☐ Definite maybe ☐

Figure answer 1-10

Rate and rhythm?	Supraventricular bradycardia at 52 bpm
Pathologic Q waves?	
ST-segment elevation?	II, III, aVF, V_3, V_5, V_6
ST-segment depression?	aVL, V_1, V_2
T-wave changes?	Inverted in aVL, V_1, V_2
Voltage criteria for LVH?	No
QRS width?	108 ms
Reciprocal changes?	aVL
STEMI?	Yes
Interpretation:	STEMI, inferolateral. ST elevation noted in II, III, aVF, V_3, V_5, and V_6. Second-degree type I AV block present, probably nodal. Does not meet voltage criteria for LVH, QRS duration within normal limits. Obvious reciprocal changes present. ST depression and tall R wave in V_1–V_2 suggestive of posterior wall involvement. As with all inferior STEMI, obtain V_4R to assess for right ventricular infarction. *Note:* ST elevation in V_3 probably due right coronary artery supplying a portion of the ventricular apex.

- PR interval 0 ms
- P-QRS-T axes 999, 62, 87
- QRS duration 108 ms
- QT/QTc 480/460 ms

Figure answer 1-11

Rate and rhythm?	Atrial fibrillation at 81 bpm
Pathologic Q waves?	
ST-segment elevation?	I, aVL
ST-segment depression?	II, III, aVF
T-wave changes?	
Voltage criteria for LVH?	No
QRS width?	92 ms
Reciprocal changes?	II, III, aVF
STEMI?	Yes
Interpretation:	STEMI, lateral. ST elevation noted in I and aVL. Does not meet voltage criteria for LVH. QRS duration within normal limits. Reciprocal changes noted in II, III and aVF.

- PR interval None
- P-QRS-T axes 999, −13, −30
- QRS duration 92 ms
- QT/QTc 388/426 ms

Figure answer 1-12

Rate and rhythm?	Sinus tachycardia at 111 bpm
Pathologic Q waves?	
ST-segment elevation?	V_1–V_3
ST-segment depression?	II, III, aVF
T-wave changes?	Tall in V_2
Voltage criteria for LVH?	No
QRS width?	92 ms
Reciprocal changes?	II, III, aVF
STEMI?	Yes
Interpretation:	STEMI, anteroseptal. ST elevation noted in V_1–V_3. Tall T waves present in V_2, borderline in V_3. Does not meet voltage criteria for LVH. QRS within normal limits. Reciprocal changes noted in II, III, and aVF.

- PR interval 192 ms
- P-QRS-T axes 63, 66, 55
- QRS duration 92 ms
- QT/QTc 328/393 ms

Figure answer 1-13

Rate and rhythm?	Sinus tachycardia at 107 bpm
Pathologic Q waves?	
ST-segment elevation?	II, III, aVF
ST-segment depression?	I, aVL
T-wave changes?	Inverted in I
Reciprocal changes?	I, aVL
STEMI?	Yes
Interpretation:	Suspected STEMI, inferior. ST depression, T-wave inversion (presumed reciprocal change) in lead aVL. T-wave inversion and slight ST depression in I.

- PR interval 192 ms
- P-QRS-T axes 75, 82, 92
- QRS duration 100 ms
- QT/QTc 332/395 ms

Figure answer 1-14

Rate and rhythm?	Sinus rhythm at 65 bpm with occasional premature complexes
Pathologic Q waves?	
ST-segment elevation?	V_2–V_5
ST-segment depression?	III, aVF
T-wave changes?	Inverted in III
Reciprocal changes?	
STEMI?	Yes
Interpretation:	Suspected STEMI, anterior.

- PR interval 140 ms
- P-QRS-T axes 62, 56, −16
- QRS duration 80 ms
- QT/QTc 396/408 ms

Figure answer 1-19

Rate and rhythm?	Sinus rhythm at 71 bpm
Pathologic Q waves?	
ST-segment elevation?	II, III, aVF
ST-segment depression?	V_2–V_4
T-wave changes?	Inverted in V_1
Voltage criteria for LVH?	No
QRS width?	108 ms
Reciprocal changes?	aVL
STEMI?	Yes
Interpretation:	STEMI, inferior. ST elevation noted in II, III, and aVF. Does not meet voltage criteria for LVH. QRS duration within normal limits. Reciprocal changes noted in aVL. Obtain V_4R to assess for RVI. ST depression in V_2–V_4 possibly from posterior involvement, consider obtaining posterior leads. Low QRS voltage in limb leads.

- PR interval 192 ms
- P-QRS-T axes 43, 44, 38
- QRS duration 108 ms
- QT/QTc 376/398 ms

Figure answer 1-20

Rate and rhythm?	Sinus rhythm at 62 bpm
Pathologic Q waves?	
ST-segment elevation?	I, aVL, V_2–V_6
ST-segment depression?	III, aVF
T-wave changes?	Tall in V_2–V_5
Voltage criteria for LVH?	Yes
QRS width?	100 ms
Reciprocal changes?	III, aVF
STEMI?	Yes
Interpretation:	STEMI, extensive anterolateral. ST elevation noted in I, aVL, V_2–V_6. QRS duration within normal limits. Clear and obvious reciprocal changes present in III and aVF. Meets minimal voltage criteria for LVH, may be normal variant.

- PR interval 192 ms
- P-QRS-T axes 66, −29, 35
- QRS duration 100 ms
- QT/QTc 388/393 ms

Figure answer 1-21

Rate and rhythm?	Sinus rhythm at 82 bpm
Pathologic Q waves?	
ST-segment elevation?	V_1-V_3
ST-segment depression?	
T-wave changes?	
Voltage criteria for LVH?	No
QRS width?	76 ms
Reciprocal changes?	No
STEMI?	Possible STEMI (definite maybe)
Interpretation:	Possible STEMI, anteroseptal. ST elevation noted in V_1-V_3. Does not meet voltage criteria for LVH. QRS duration within normal limits. No reciprocal changes noted. This DOES NOT rule out STEMI. Remember, not all STEMI produce reciprocal changes. However, without reciprocal changes, BER and pericarditis remain possible explanations for ST elevation. In addition, slight ST elevation in V_1-V_3 can be a normal variant (high takeoff). As always, consider clinical presentation and use ST trending or serial ECGs.

- PR interval 168 ms
- P-QRS-T axes 68, 67, 38
- QRS duration 76 ms
- QT/QTc 356/395 ms

REFERENCE

1. Wagner GS, Macfarlane P, Wellens H, et al. AHA/ACCF/HRS recommendations for the standardization and interpretation of the electrocardiogram: part VI: acute ischemia/infarction: a scientific statement from the American Heart Association Electrocardiography and Arrhythmias Committee, Council on Clinical Cardiology; the American College of Cardiology Foundation; and the Heart Rhythm Society, *J Am Coll Cardiol* 53:1003–1011, 2009.

STEMI Imposters

aVR   V1

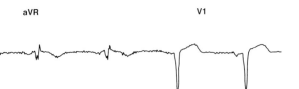

STEMI is not the only cause of ST elevation. In fact, other noninfarct causes of ST elevation are common. We will call them the STEMI imposters. The top STEMI imposters are listed in Box 2-1.

Think of it this way: The two main causes of ST elevation are STEMI and the STEMI imposters. If you can eliminate the top STEMI imposters as the cause of the ST elevation on a 12-lead ECG, that leaves you with STEMI as the most likely cause. It is important to note that the approach offered in this chapter will not work 100% of the time. Rather, it works in the majority of cases, probably around 90% of the time. In reality, anyone reading this quick guide is not the person who will "pull the trigger" and make the final decision on who gets reperfused. Instead, our job is most likely to maximize the number of STEMIs identified at first contact with a reasonable number of false positives.

If you were only interested in maximizing the number of STEMIs identified at first contact, then you could call a STEMI alert on every patient you encounter. Obviously, that is ridiculous and you would have an unacceptable number of false-positive STEMI activations, but you would not miss any.

Box 2-1	STEMI Imposters

- Left ventricular hypertrophy
- Bundle branch block
- Ventricular rhythms
- Benign early repolarization
- Pericarditis

Conversely, if you were most interested in eliminating false positives, then you might only call STEMI when you were 100% sure with no doubts or questions whatsoever. The problem with this strategy is that many people who could have benefited from immediate reperfusion would not have received it in a timely manner because you were overly hesitant to call it a STEMI.

Key Point

STEMI Recognition – Goal # 2:
When you say the ST elevation found is caused by STEMI, you are right 9 times out of 10.

Achieving balance is the key. One could err by being too quick to call STEMI and ignoring the STEMI imposters. One could also err by being overly concerned about the STEMI imposters. Our assumption is that when you call STEMI, if you are right 90% of the time, you are approaching the sweet spot for maximizing the number of STEMIs identified with an acceptable number of false positives. This chapter intends to provide a simple strategy to help you achieve that balance.

We will examine the top STEMI imposters, describe the ECG findings associated with each, and provide a strategy that can be used to try and eliminate them as possible causes of the ST elevation. We will start with left ventricular hypertrophy.

Left Ventricular Hypertrophy

Left ventricular hypertrophy (LVH) refers to enlargement of the left ventricle. The left ventricle can enlarge for a variety of reasons, such as uncontrolled hypertension. Whatever the cause, if the left ventricle is enlarged the patient may have ST elevation on the resting ECG.

LVH is recognized by increased QRS amplitude. That is, LVH tends to produce QRS complexes that are in some leads taller and in other leads deeper. Many formulas exist to try and recognize LVH. Some of them are quite sophisticated and difficult to memorize. The formula presented here was selected because it is easy to remember and may be used to quickly check for the presence of LVH.

Step 1
- Look at V_1 and determine the depth of the S wave by counting in millimeters the amount of negative deflection measuring from the baseline to the most negative point in V_1 (count the small boxes—one box equals 1 mm).

Step 2
- Look at V_5 and V_6 and determine which lead has the tallest R wave.
- Determine the height of the taller R wave in millimeters (count the small boxes).

Step 3
- Add the height of the taller R wave and the deeper S wave.
- If the number is equal to or greater than 35, suspect LVH.

If ST elevation is present, and the ECG *did not* meet the voltage criteria for LVH, then it is reasonable to assume the elevation noted was not caused by LVH. One imposter down, four to go.

Bundle Branch Block and Ventricular Rhythms

Bundle branch blocks (BBBs) and ventricular rhythms (including paced ventricular rhythms) can be easily scratched off the list of STEMI imposters. Both of these entities produce a wide

QRS complex (120 ms or more). If the QRS is narrow, then neither a complete BBB nor ventricular rhythm is present.

The easiest way to determine the QRS duration is to let the machine measure it for you. If the QRS duration is less than 120 ms, then any ST elevation that is present is assumed to be the result of a cause other than a complete BBB or ventricular rhythm.

Benign Early Repolarization and Pericarditis

Benign early repolarization (BER) is a normal variant that produces an ECG pattern with changes very similar to STEMI. For example, BER may produce ST elevation and tall T waves.

Pericarditis, an inflamed pericardium, may also produce ST elevation. If all of the pericardium is inflamed, then the ST elevation may be in present in all or most of the ECG leads. Or, if not occurring in all of the leads, the ST elevation may be noted in leads that are not normally grouped together. There is also a classic clinical presentation that includes chest pain. So this can be a tricky call.

The point to be made here is not to rule out an acute MI but rather to exclude pericarditis or BER as a cause of ST elevation. While both BER and pericarditis can cause ST elevation, neither produces obvious reciprocal changes. So, if reciprocal changes are present, neither BER or pericarditis is likely to be the cause of the ST elevation.

The answers to three questions will determine if you can eliminate the top STEMI imposters as the cause of ST elevation.

The three questions are:
1. Is the voltage criteria met for LVH?
2. What is the QRS duration?
3. Are reciprocal changes present?

If the voltage criterion for LVH is not met, then LVH is not producing the ST elevation. If the QRS is less than 120 ms, then BBB and ventricular rhythms are not the cause of the ST segment elevation. If reciprocal changes are present, then you can reasonably eliminate BER and pericarditis as causes of the elevation.

We can now fully describe the five-step approach for STEMI recognition:

Step 1. Identify the rate and underlying rhythm.

Step 2. Analyze waveforms. Examine each lead (except aVR), looking for these five key waveform changes:
- Pathologic Q waves
- ST-segment elevation
- ST-segment depression
- Tall, peaked T waves
- Inverted T waves

Step 3. Examine for evidence of infarction. Suspected STEMI? Location?

Step 4. Ascertain if STEMI imposters are present that may account for ECG changes.
- Voltage criteria for LVH?
- QRS duration?
- Reciprocal changes?

Step 5. Make a STEMI decision. We suggest using a simple three-part question to decide whether a STEMI is present based on your ECG findings:
- *A STEMI is definitely not present.* No STEMI means that ST elevation of 1 mm or more in at least two anatomically contiguous leads was not present. Remember, the patient could be experiencing an acute MI, but if there is no ST elevation, there is no STEMI. Treat the patient per appropriate protocols and obtain serial ECGs or use ST-segment monitoring. It is possible that this ECG did not have ST elevation but a future ECG might.
- *A suspected STEMI is present.* This category is for those patients whose ECGs meet the ST elevation criteria for STEMI *and* you have eliminated the top STEMI imposters as possible causes of the elevation. There is not a 100% guarantee that STEMI is present, but with the appropriate clinical

presentation, you should be right about 9 times out of 10.

- *A STEMI may or may not be present (definite maybe).* When the ST segment is elevated and a STEMI imposter is also present it can be difficult to determine the precise cause of that elevation—STEMI or STEMI imposter? Although the patient's clinical presentation is a key component in the decision, in many cases it will still be a very difficult determination to make. Therefore when the ECG is equivocal for STEMI or a STEMI imposter, call it a possible STEMI. Serial ECGs and ST-segment monitoring can help solve the mystery. So can passing the ECG along for review by a more experienced interpreter. It is best to know in advance what your EMS system or facility wants you to do when you suspect a STEMI clinically, find ST-segment elevation on the patient's ECG, and recognize that a STEMI imposter exists.

Review the following practice ECGs (Figures 2-1 through 2-5) using the five-step approach and categorize each as: No STEMI, Suspected STEMI, or Possible STEMI.

PRACTICE ECGs

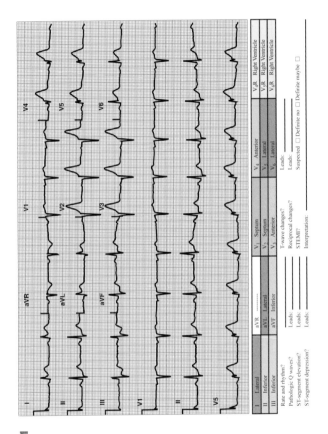

Figure 2-1

	I	Lateral	aVR		V₁	Septum	V₄	Anterior	V₄R	Right Ventricle
	II	Inferior	aVL	Lateral	V₂	Septum	V₅	Lateral	V₅R	Right Ventricle
	III	Inferior	aVF	Inferior	V₃	Anterior	V₆	Lateral	V₆R	Right Ventricle

Rate and rhythm: _____
Pathologic Q waves?   Leads: _____
ST-segment elevation?   Leads: _____
ST-segment depression?   Leads: _____

T-wave changes? _____
Reciprocal changes? _____
STEMI?   Suspected ☐ Definite no ☐ Definite maybe ☐
Interpretation: _____

Figure 2-2

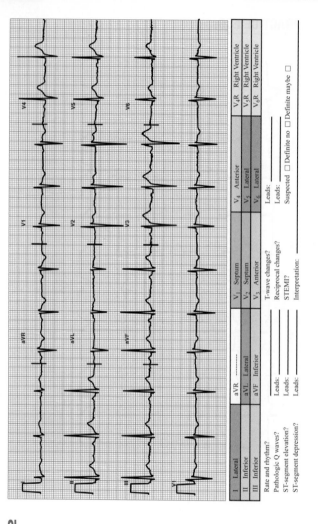

I	Lateral	aVR	---------	V₁	Septum	V₄	Anterior	V₄R	Right Ventricle
II	Inferior	aVL	Lateral	V₂	Septum	V₅	Lateral	V₅R	Right Ventricle
III	Inferior	aVF	Inferior	V₃	Anterior	V₆	Lateral	V₆R	Right Ventricle

Rate and rhythm?

Pathologic Q waves?   Leads:

ST-segment elevation?   Leads:

ST-segment depression?   Leads:

T-wave changes?

Reciprocal changes?   Leads: _____

STEMI?   Leads: _____

Suspected ☐ Definite no ☐ Definite maybe ☐

Interpretation: _____

Figure 2-3

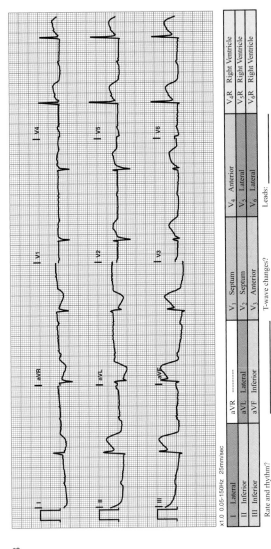

x1.0 0.05-150Hz 25mm/sec							
I	Lateral	aVR	-------	V₁	Septum	V₄	Anterior	V₄R	Right Ventricle
II	Inferior	aVL	Lateral	V₂	Septum	V₅	Lateral	V₅R	Right Ventricle
III	Inferior	aVF	Inferior	V₃	Anterior	V₆	Lateral	V₆R	Right Ventricle

Rate and rhythm? _____

Pathologic Q waves? Leads: _____

ST-segment elevation? Leads: _____

ST-segment depression? Leads: _____

T-wave changes? _____

Reciprocal changes? _____

STEMI? Leads: _____

       Leads: _____

Suspected ☐ Definite no ☐ Definite maybe ☐

Interpretation: _____

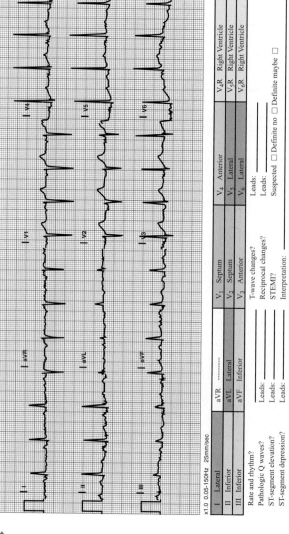

x1.0 0.05-150Hz 25mm/sec

I	Lateral	aVR	---------	V$_1$	Septum	V$_4$R	Right Ventricle
II	Inferior	aVL	Lateral	V$_2$	Septum	V$_5$R	Right Ventricle
III	Inferior	aVF	Inferior	V$_3$	Anterior	V$_6$R	Right Ventricle

		V$_4$	Anterior
		V$_5$	Lateral
		V$_6$	Lateral

Rate and rhythm? _____
Pathologic Q waves?   Leads: _____   T-wave changes? _____   Leads: _____
ST-segment elevation?   Leads: _____   Reciprocal changes? _____   Leads: _____
ST-segment depression?   Leads: _____   STEMI? _____   Suspected ☐ Definite no ☐ Definite maybe ☐
   Interpretation: _____

Figure 2-4

Figure 2-5

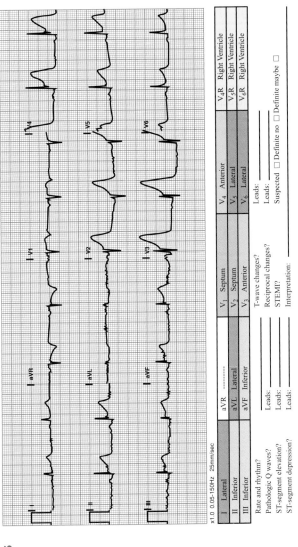

x1.0 0.05-150Hz 25mm/sec

I Lateral	aVR -------	V₁ Septum	V₄ Anterior	V₄R Right Ventricle
II Inferior	aVL Lateral	V₂ Septum	V₅ Lateral	V₅R Right Ventricle
III Inferior	aVF Inferior	V₃ Anterior	V₆ Lateral	V₆R Right Ventricle

Rate and rhythm? _____

Pathologic Q waves? Leads: _____

ST-segment elevation? Leads: _____

ST-segment depression? Leads: _____

T-wave changes? _____

Reciprocal changes? _____

STEMI? Leads: _____

Interpretation: _____

Suspected ☐ Definite no ☐ Definite maybe ☐

PRACTICE ECGs–INTERPRETATIONS

Figure answer 2-1

Rate and rhythm?	Sinus bradycardia at 58 bpm
Pathologic Q waves?	
ST-segment elevation?	I, aVL, V_2–V_6
ST-segment depression?	II, III, aVF
T-wave changes?	
Voltage criteria for LVH?	No
QRS width?	92 ms
Reciprocal changes?	II, III, aVF
STEMI?	Yes
Interpretation:	STEMI, extensive anterolateral. ST elevation noted in I, aVL, V_2–V_6. Does not meet voltage criteria for LVH. QRS duration within normal limits. Obvious reciprocal changes in II, III, and aVF.

- PR interval 184 ms
- P-QRS-T axes 39, 16, 16
- QRS duration 92 ms
- QT/QTc 416/409 ms

Figure answer 2-2

Rate and rhythm?	Sinus rhythm at 67 bpm with right bundle branch block
Pathologic Q waves?	
ST-segment elevation?	V₃
ST-segment depression?	
T-wave changes?	
Voltage criteria for LVH?	No
QRS width?	108 ms
Reciprocal changes?	No
STEMI?	No
Interpretation:	No ECG evidence of STEMI noted. Incomplete RBBB pattern, may be normal variant for young male.

Rate and rhythm? — Sinus rhythm at 67 bpm with right bundle branch block

ST-segment elevation? — V_3

Voltage criteria for LVH? — No

QRS width? — 108 ms

Reciprocal changes? — No

STEMI? — No

Interpretation: — No ECG evidence of STEMI noted. Incomplete RBBB pattern, may be normal variant for young male.

- PR interval 158 ms
- P-QRS-T axes 71, 83, 71
- QRS duration 108 ms
- QT/QTc 400/422 ms

Figure answer 2-3

Rate and rhythm?	Supraventricular bradycardia at 42 bpm
Pathologic Q waves?	
ST-segment elevation?	II, III, aVF, V_2–V_6
ST-segment depression?	I, aVL
T-wave changes?	
Voltage criteria for LVH?	No
QRS width?	92 ms
Reciprocal changes?	I, aVL
STEMI?	Yes
Interpretation:	STEMI, inferolateral. ST elevation notes in II, III, aVF, V_5, and V_6. Tall T waves seen in II, III and aVF. Does not meet he voltage criteria for LVH. QRS within normal limits. Obvious reciprocal changes noted in I and aVL. Obtain V_4R to assess for RVI.

- PR interval 0 ms
- P-QRS-T axes 999, 69, 94
- QRS duration 92 ms
- QT/QTc 516/460 ms

Figure answer 2-4

Rate and rhythm?	Sinus rhythm at 89 bpm
Pathologic Q waves?	
ST-segment elevation?	
ST-segment depression?	
T-wave changes?	
Voltage criteria for LVH?	No
QRS width?	84 ms
Reciprocal changes?	No
STEMI?	No
Interpretation:	Nonspecific T-wave abnormality; baseline wander in V_5–V_6. No ECG evidence of STEMI. As always, consider clinical presentation and use ST trending or serial ECGs.

- PR interval 184 ms
- P-QRS-T axes 54, 45, 75
- QRS duration 84 ms
- QT/QTc 348/395 ms

Figure answer 2-5

Rate and rhythm?	Sinus bradycardia at 55 bpm
Pathologic Q waves?	
ST-segment elevation?	II, III, aVF, V_2–V_6
ST-segment depression?	aVL
T-wave changes?	Tall in II, aVF, V_2–V_4
Voltage criteria for LVH?	No
QRS width?	84 ms
Reciprocal changes?	aVL
STEMI?	Yes
Interpretation:	STEMI, global. ST elevation noted in II, III, aVF, V_2–V_6. Tall T waves present in II, aVF, V_2–V_4. Voltage criteria for LVH not met. QRS duration within normal limits. With such widespread ST elevation, pericarditis is always a consideration. In this case, the ST depression in aVL (the lead most likely to show a reciprocal change with inferior STEMI) suggests STEMI. As always, considered clinical presentation and use ST trending or serial ECGs.

- PR interval 176 ms
- P-QRS-T axes 75, 58, 66
- QRS duration 84 ms
- QT/QTc 444/433 ms

Additional Lead ECGs

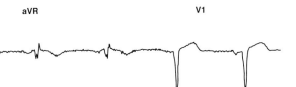

As good as the 12-lead ECG is, it is not perfect. Among its shortcomings is that it has two "blind spots." The 12-lead ECG does not see the right ventricle, nor does it directly view the posterior wall of the left ventricle. That makes sense considering the 12-lead was around for decades before it was used for STEMI recognition. Since it was not designed for STEMI recognition, it is no surprise that it does not do the job perfectly.

To overcome this, you can learn when it would be advisable to obtain additional leads, how to use your existing equipment to obtain them, and how to interpret these additional leads. In this chapter, we discuss the right ventricle, the posterior wall, and end with a discussion of 15- and 18-lead ECGs, which simply are standard 12-leads along with some additional leads to view the right ventricle and posterior wall.

Key Point

STEMI Recognition – Goal # 3:
You know when and how to use additional leads for STEMI recognition.

Right Ventricle

As shown in Figure 3-1, the blood supply to the inferior wall of the left ventricle is provided by the right coronary artery in most patients. The right ventricle is also supplied by the right coronary artery. Therefore when an inferior STEMI is present, if the occlusion in the right coronary artery is proximal, the right ventricle can be affected as well.

Right ventricular infarction (RVI) is not infrequent. When an inferior STEMI is present, the right ventricle is also infarcting about 40% of the time. Because the standard 12-lead does not see the right ventricle, it may not be obvious from the 12-lead obtained which inferior STEMI patients have an occlusion proximal enough in the right coronary artery to affect the right ventricle.

If an electrode and lead wire, however, were to be placed on the right chest, then it would be possible to "view" the right ventricle. This lead could be examined for ST elevation and, if found, RVI would be suspected. *At a minimum, obtain at least one right-sided chest lead every time you suspect inferior STEMI.* If ST elevation is found in the right-sided chest lead, then you should suspect that the right ventricle is also infarcting.

Leads V_3R through V_6R have the same placement as their counterpart on the standard 12-lead, except they are positioned in the symmetrically opposite position on the right side of the chest. Figure 3-2 and Table 3-1 show and explain the position of the right chest leads.

RVI identifies a patient who is sensitive to changes in preload. Remember that the right ventricle's job is to pump blood through the lungs to the left side of the heart. If the right ventricle is infarcting, it may not be able to do its job as well. This could result in a reduction in left ventricular filling, or preload. If an RVI is suspected, be aware that any drug that reduces preload has the potential to produce a significant drop in blood pressure. Conversely, if the patient's blood pressure is already low, improving preload is probably the treatment he or she will respond to best.

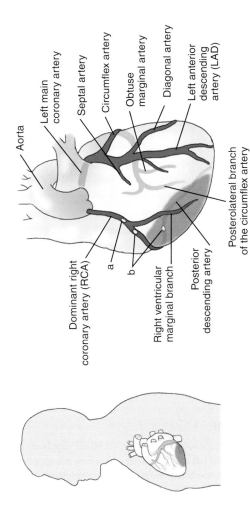

Figure 3-1 Inferior wall infarction. Coronary anatomy shows a dominant right coronary artery (RCA). Occlusion at point "A" results in an inferior and right ventricular infarction. Occlusion at point "B" is limited to the inferior wall, sparing the right ventricle.

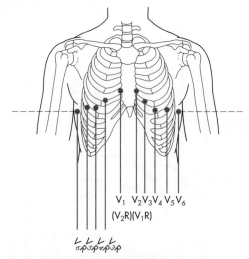

Figure 3-2 Anatomic placement of the left and right chest leads.

Table 3-1	Right Chest Leads and Their Placement
Lead	Placement
V₁R	Lead V₂
V₂R	Lead V₁
V₃R	Midway between V₂R and V₄R
V₄R	Right midclavicular line, fifth intercostal space
V₅R	Right anterior axillary line at same level as V₄R
V₆R	Right midaxillary line at same level as V₄R

Posterior Wall

The posterior (inferobasal) wall may get its blood supply from either the right or the left coronary artery, but often it is supplied by both. Therefore, posterior infarction can complicate both inferior STEMI and lateral STEMI. The real issue occurs when the posterior wall is experiencing an isolated STEMI. When this occurs (the posterior wall is infarcting "all by itself"), there will be no ST elevation noted on the standard 12-lead ECG. This patient could benefit from reperfusion, but the isolated posterior STEMI must first be identified!

To identify a posterior STEMI, electrodes and lead cables are moved to the back of the left chest. From there the new leads can "see" the posterior wall. These new leads can then be examined for the presence of ST elevation.

Electrode Placement

Three possible posterior leads can be obtained. They continue on the horizontal plane formed by V_4–V_6. The posterior leads are V_7–V_9. Lead V_7 is placed at the posterior axillary line. Lead V_8 is placed at the angle of the scapula (posterior scapular line), and lead V_9 is placed over the left border of the spine. Figure 3-3 shows the position of the posterior chest leads.

Lead Cable Placement

Any of the chest lead cables (V_1–V_6) can be moved to obtain any additional chest lead. So there is no single "right way" for which chest cable gets a specific additional chest lead. Practically speaking, though, there may be some cable configurations that are easier to use than others. Once the additional leads have been obtained, you will need to relabel them accordingly. Also, disregard the interpretive statement since the device has no idea you have moved the cables. Last, if you transmit ECGs, either do not transmit the additional leads (your relabeling will not be transmitted) or use a comments field to identify the additional leads.

Key Point

Fifteen- and 18-lead ECGs are being used with increasing frequency to help spot infarctions of the right ventricle and the posterior wall of the left ventricle. The 15-lead ECG uses all leads of a standard 12-lead plus leads V_4R, V_8, and V_9. An 18-lead ECG uses the 15-lead ECG plus leads V_5R, V_6R, and V_7.

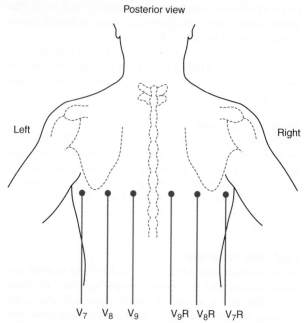

Figure 3-3 Posterior chest leads are used when a posterior infarction is suspected. Leads V$_7$, V$_8$, and V$_9$ are on the same horizontal line as leads V$_4$, V$_5$, and V$_6$ on the front of the chest. Lead V$_7$ is placed at the posterior axillary line. Lead V$_8$ is placed at the angle of the scapula (posterior scapular line) and lead V$_9$ is placed over the left border of the spine.

Interpretation

The complexes obtained in the additional leads are often smaller than the complexes in the standard 12-leads. The reason that the right-sided complexes are smaller is because the right ventricle has significantly less mass than does the left ventricle. The reason the posterior leads are smaller is due to the fact that the heart is positioned more anteriorly in the chest and the posterior leads have to "look" though more tissue, so to speak.

The fact the QRS complexes are smaller in the additional leads brings up the question, "Do we need to see less ST elevation in the additional leads to suspect STEMI?" While there is no clear-cut answer from the STEMI Guidelines, many believe that 0.5 mm of elevation in the additional leads is suggestive of STEMI.

Because ST elevation in two contiguous leads is required when identifying STEMI, individuals often ask, "Why don't you need two right-sided leads?" The answer is that if an inferior STEMI is what prompted you to look for an RVI, then you already have elevation in two contiguous leads. You are only obtaining V_4R to see how far the STEMI extends; thus, one is sufficient. However, when looking for an isolated STEMI (either isolated posterior or isolated right ventricular), be sure to have at least two leads displaying ST elevation before claiming STEMI to be present.

Practice ECGs

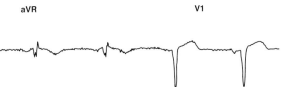

aVR V1

Here are 10 ECGs for you to practice the five-step approach previously discussed (Box 4-1). As you go through Figures 4-1 through 4-10, consider which of these ECGs might prompt you to obtain additional leads. Remember: there are over 100 practice ECGs in *The 12-Lead ECG in Acute Coronary Syndromes* textbook. Good luck!

Box **4-1**	Summary of the Five-Step Approach to 12-Lead Analysis and STEMI Recognition

Step 1: Rate and rhythm

Step 2: Look for evidence of STEMI
  Pathologic Q wave
  ST elevation
  ST depression
  Tall T wave
  Inverted T wave

Step 3: Suspect STEMI?
  If so, where?

Step 4: STEMI Imposters?
  Voltage criteria for LVH?
  QRS duration?
  Reciprocal changes?

Step 5: Categorize ECG
  No STEMI
  Suspected STEMI
  Possible STEMI

Figure 4-1

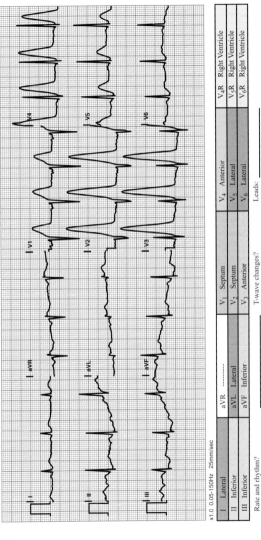

x1.0 0.05-150Hz 25mm/sec

I Lateral	aVR ------	V₁ Septum	V₄ Anterior	V₄R Right Ventricle
II Inferior	aVL Lateral	V₂ Septum	V₅ Lateral	V₅R Right Ventricle
III Inferior	aVF Inferior	V₃ Anterior	V₆ Lateral	V₆R Right Ventricle

Rate and rhythm? _____

Pathologic Q waves?   Leads: _____   T-wave changes?   Leads: _____

ST-segment elevation?   Leads: _____   Reciprocal changes?   Leads: _____

ST-segment depression?   Leads: _____   STEMI?   Suspected ☐ Definite no ☐ Definite maybe ☐

Interpretation: _____

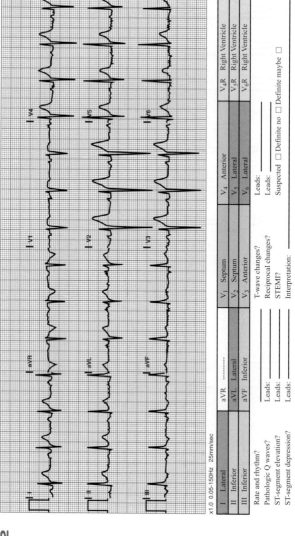

x1.0 0.05-150Hz 25mm/sec

I	Lateral	aVR	---------	V₁	Septum	V₄	Anterior	V₄R	Right Ventricle
II	Inferior	aVL	Lateral	V₂	Septum	V₅	Lateral	V₅R	Right Ventricle
III	Inferior	aVF	Inferior	V₃	Anterior	V₆	Lateral	V₆R	Right Ventricle

Rate and rhythm? _____

Pathologic Q waves? _____ Leads: _____

ST-segment elevation? _____ Leads: _____

ST-segment depression? _____ Leads: _____

T-wave changes? _____ Leads: _____

Reciprocal changes? _____ Leads: _____

STEMI? _____ Suspected ☐ Definite no ☐ Definite maybe ☐

Interpretation: _____

Figure 4-2

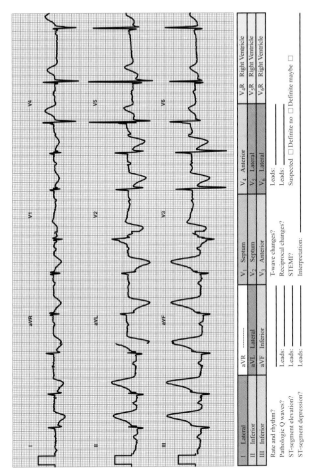

I	Lateral	aVR	------	V₁	Septum	V₄	Anterior	V₄R	Right Ventricle
II	Inferior	aVL	Lateral	V₂	Septum	V₅	Lateral	V₅R	Right Ventricle
III	Inferior	aVF	Inferior	V₃	Anterior	V₆	Lateral	V₆R	Right Ventricle

Rate and rhythm? _____

Pathologic Q waves? Leads: _____

ST-segment elevation? Leads: _____

ST-segment depression? Leads: _____

T-wave changes? Leads: _____

Reciprocal changes? Leads: _____

STEMI? Suspected ☐ Definite no ☐ Definite maybe ☐

Interpretation: _____

Figure 4-3

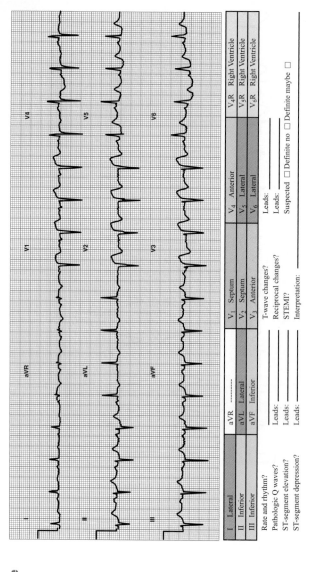

I Lateral	aVR --------	V$_1$ Septum	V$_4$R Right Ventricle
II Inferior	aVL Lateral	V$_2$ Septum	V$_5$R Right Ventricle
III Inferior	aVF Inferior	V$_3$ Anterior	V$_6$R Right Ventricle

| | | V$_4$ Anterior | |
| V$_5$ Lateral |
| V$_6$ Lateral |

Rate and rhythm? _____

Pathologic Q waves? Leads: _____   T-wave changes? Leads: _____

ST-segment elevation? Leads: _____   Reciprocal changes? Leads: _____

ST-segment depression? Leads: _____   STEM? Suspected ☐ Definite no ☐ Definite maybe ☐

Interpretation: _____

Figure 4-4

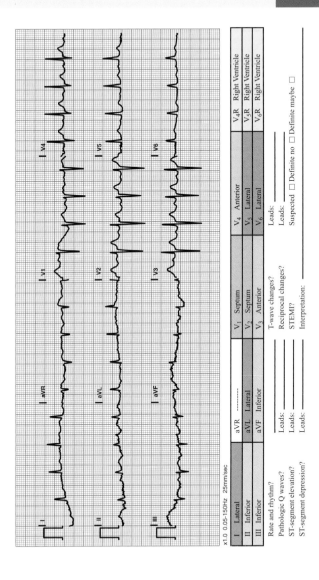

x1.0 0.05–150Hz   25mm/sec

I Lateral	aVR		V1 Septum	V4 Anterior	V4R Right Ventricle
II Inferior	aVL Lateral		V2 Septum	V5 Lateral	V5R Right Ventricle
III Inferior	aVF Inferior		V3 Anterior	V6 Lateral	V6R Right Ventricle

Rate and rhythm? _____
Pathologic Q waves? _____ Leads: _____
ST-segment elevation? _____ Leads: _____
ST-segment depression? _____ Leads: _____

T-wave changes? _____
Reciprocal changes? _____ Leads: _____
STEMI? _____ Leads: _____
Interpretation: _____

Suspected ☐ Definite no ☐ Definite maybe ☐

Figure
4-5

Figure 4-6

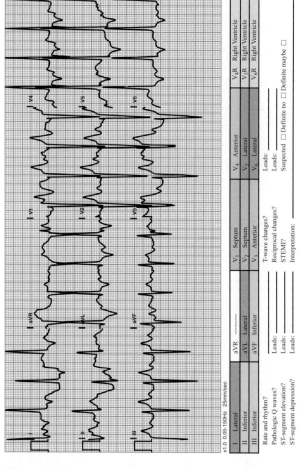

x1.0 0.05-150Hz 25mv/sec

I Lateral	aVR ---------	V₁ Septum	V₄ Anterior	V₄R Right Ventricle
II Inferior	aVL Lateral	V₂ Septum	V₅ Lateral	V₅R Right Ventricle
III Inferior	aVF Inferior	V₃ Anterior	V₆ Lateral	V₆R Right Ventricle

Rate and rhythm?

Pathologic Q waves? _____   T-wave changes? _____   Leads: _____

ST-segment elevation? _____   Reciprocal changes? _____   Leads: _____

ST-segment depression? _____   STEMI? _____

Leads: _____   Interpretation: _____   Suspected □ Definite no □ Definite maybe □

Figure 4-7

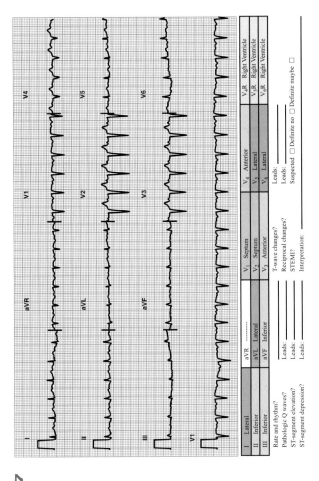

I Lateral	aVR	V₁ Septum	V₄ Anterior	V₄R Right Ventricle
II Inferior	aVL Lateral	V₂ Septum	V₅ Lateral	V₅R Right Ventricle
III Inferior	aVF Inferior	V₃ Anterior	V₆ Lateral	V₆R Right Ventricle

Rate and rhythm? _____

Pathologic Q waves? Leads: _____ T-wave changes? Leads: _____

ST-segment elevation? Leads: _____ Reciprocal changes? Leads: _____

ST-segment depression? Leads: _____ STEMI? Suspected ☐ Definite no ☐ Definite maybe ☐

Interpretation: _____

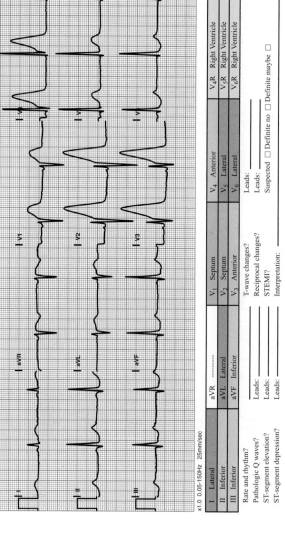

x1.0 0.05-150Hz 25mm/sec

I	Lateral	aVR	--------	V₁	Septum	V₄	Anterior	V₄R	Right Ventricle
II	Inferior	aVL	Lateral	V₂	Septum	V₅	Lateral	V₅R	Right Ventricle
III	Inferior	aVF	Inferior	V₃	Anterior	V₆	Lateral	V₆R	Right Ventricle

Rate and rhythm? _____

Pathologic Q waves? Leads: _____   T-wave changes? _____   Leads: _____

ST-segment elevation? Leads: _____   Reciprocal changes? _____   Leads: _____

ST-segment depression? Leads: _____   STEMI? Suspected ☐ Definite ☐ Definite no ☐ Definite maybe ☐

Interpretation: _____

Figure 4-8

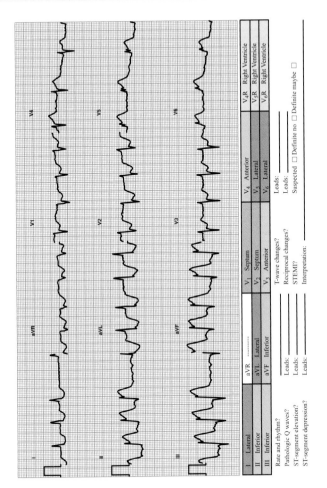

Figure 4-9

I	Lateral	aVR	---------	V₁	Septum	V₄	Anterior	V₄R	Right Ventricle
II	Inferior	aVL	Lateral	V₂	Septum	V₅	Lateral	V₅R	Right Ventricle
III	Inferior	aVF	Inferior	V₃	Anterior	V₆	Lateral	V₆R	Right Ventricle

Rate and rhythm? _____   T-wave changes? _____

Pathologic Q waves? _____   Reciprocal changes? _____   Leads: _____

ST-segment elevation? _____ Leads: _____   STEMI? _____   Leads: _____

ST-segment depression? _____ Leads: _____   Interpretation: _____   Suspected ☐ Definite no ☐ Definite maybe ☐

Figure 4-10

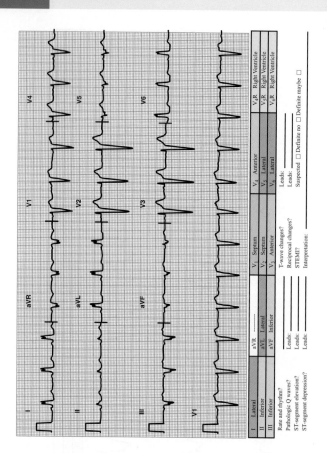

I Lateral	aVR --------	V₁ Septum	V₄ Anterior	V₄R Right Ventricle
II Inferior	aVL Lateral	V₂ Septum	V₅ Lateral	V₅R Right Ventricle
III Inferior	aVF Inferior	V₃ Anterior	V₆ Lateral	V₆R Right Ventricle

Rate and rhythm: _____
Pathologic Q waves? _____   T-wave changes? _____
ST-segment elevation? _____   Reciprocal changes? _____
ST-segment depression? _____   STEMI? _____
Leads: _____   Leads: _____
Leads: _____   Leads: _____
Leads: _____   Suspected □ Definite no □ Definite maybe □
          Interpretation: _____

PRACTICE ECGs—INTERPRETATIONS

Figure answer 4-1

Rate and rhythm?	Sinus rhythm at 81 bpm
Pathologic Q waves?	
ST-segment elevation?	aVL, V_1–V_4
ST-segment depression?	II, III, aVF
T-wave changes?	Inverted in III, tall in V_1–V_4
Voltage criteria for LVH?	No
QRS width?	88 ms
Reciprocal changes?	II, III, aVF
STEMI?	Suspected STEMI
Interpretation:	STEMI, anteroseptal. ST elevation noted in V_1–V_4 (aVL suspicious but ECG quality makes it difficult to be certain). Tall, peaked T waves seen in V_2–V_4. Does not meet voltage criteria for LVH. QRS duration within normal limits. Reciprocal changes in II, III, and aVF. Baseline wander in most limb leads.

- PR interval 144 ms
- P-QRS-T axes 55, 59, −3
- QRS duration 88 ms
- QT/QTc 372/410 ms

Figure answer 4-2

Rate and rhythm?	Sinus rhythm at 82 bpm
Pathologic Q waves?	
ST-segment elevation?	V_1–V_3
ST-segment depression?	
T-wave changes?	Inverted in III, tall in V_2–V_3
Voltage criteria for LVH?	No
QRS width?	96 ms
Reciprocal changes?	No
STEMI?	No
Interpretation:	No ECG evidence of STEMI. Borderline ST elevation in V_1–V_3 range, especially in V_2. Close but does not appear to meet ST criteria at this time. As always, consider clinical presentation and use ST trending or serial ECGs.

- PR interval 188 ms
- P-QRS-T axes −11, 76, 17
- QRS duration 96 ms
- QT/QTc 336/375 ms

Figure answer 4-3

Rate and rhythm?	Sinus rhythm with first-degree AV block at 66 bpm with occasional supraventricular premature complexes
Pathologic Q waves?	II, III, aVF
ST-segment elevation?	II, III, aVF
ST-segment depression?	I, aVL
T-wave changes?	Tall in II, III, aVF
Voltage criteria for LVH?	No
QRS width?	104 ms
Reciprocal changes?	I, aVL
STEMI?	Yes
Interpretation:	STEMI, inferior. ST elevation, tall T waves, and pathologic Q waves noted in II, III, and aVF. Does not meet voltage criteria for LVH. QRS indicates abnormal ventricular conduction but duration is within normal limits. Obvious reciprocal changes noted in I and aVL. ST depression and T-wave inversion in V_2 and V_3 suggest possible posterior involvement, consider obtaining posterior chest leads. Obtain V_4R to assess for RVI.

- PR interval 260 ms
- P-QRS-T axes 90, −75, 105
- QRS duration 104 ms
- QT/QTc444/458 ms

Figure answer 4-4

Rate and rhythm?	Sinus rhythm at 95 bpm
Pathologic Q waves?	V_2
ST-segment elevation?	V_1–V_3
ST-segment depression?	
T-wave changes?	Inverted in aVL
Voltage criteria for LVH?	No
QRS width?	96 ms
Reciprocal changes?	No
STEMI?	Yes
Interpretation:	STEMI, anteroseptal (if clinical picture suggests acute MI). Baseline wander V_5–V_6. ST elevation noted in V_1–V_3 and T-wave inversion suggest possible STEMI. However, QS complex in V_2 and poor R wave progression through V_4 make previous MI with persistent ST elevation a distinct possibility. As always, consider clinical presentation and use ST trending or serial ECGs.

- PR interval 164 ms
- P-QRS-T axes 62, −62, 83
- QRS duration 96 ms
- QT/QTc 380/433 ms

Figure answer 4-5

Rate and rhythm?	Sinus tachycardia at 108 bpm
Pathologic Q waves?	
ST-segment elevation?	
ST-segment depression?	V_5–V_6
T-wave changes?	
Voltage criteria for LVH?	No
QRS width?	80 ms
Reciprocal changes?	No
STEMI?	No
Interpretation:	Nonspecific T-wave abnormality. Baseline wander in I, III, aVL, aVF, and V_1. No ECG evidence of STEMI noted. As always, consider clinical presentation and use ST trending or serial ECGs.

- PR interval 124 ms
- P-QRS-T axes −22, 4, 65
- QRS duration 80 ms
- QT/QTc 312/375 ms

Figure answer 4-6

Rate and rhythm?	Supraventricular rhythm at 91 bpm
Pathologic Q waves?	
ST-segment elevation?	V_1-V_3
ST-segment depression?	I, II, aVL, V_4-V_6
T-wave changes?	Inverted in I, aVL, V_4-V_6
Voltage criteria for LVH?	Yes
QRS width?	108 ms
Reciprocal changes?	No
STEMI?	Possible STEMI (definite maybe)
Interpretation:	Possible STEMI. Poor ECG quality but appears ST elevation is present in V_1-V_3. However, the voltage criteria for LVH are also met. As always, consider clinical presentation and use ST trending or serial ECGs.

- PR interval 0 ms
- P-QRS-T axes 999, −14, 145
- QRS duration 108 ms
- QT/QTc 348/396 ms

Figure answer 4-7

Rate and rhythm?	Sinus tachycardia at 136 bpm
Pathologic Q waves?	V$_1$–V$_4$
ST-segment elevation?	
ST-segment depression?	
T-wave changes?	
Voltage criteria for LVH?	No
QRS width?	86 ms
Reciprocal changes?	No
STEMI?	No
Interpretation:	No ECG evidence of STEMI. Low voltage QRS; baseline wander I, III, V$_6$. As always, consider clinical presentation and use ST trending or serial ECGs.

- PR interval 146 ms
- P-QRS-T axes 42, 48, 29
- QRS duration 86 ms
- QT/QTc 278/418 ms

Figure answer 4-8

Rate and rhythm?	Sinus bradycardia at 56 bpm with short PR interval
Pathologic Q waves?	
ST-segment elevation?	V_1–V_4
ST-segment depression?	II, III, aVF
T-wave changes?	Tall in V_2–V_4
Voltage criteria for LVH?	No
QRS width?	100 ms
Reciprocal changes?	II, III, aVF
STEMI?	Yes
Interpretation:	Suspected STEMI, anteroseptal. ST elevation noted in V_1–V_4. Does not meet voltage criteria for LVH. QRS within normal limits. Reciprocal changes noted in II, III and aVF.

- PR interval 116 ms
- P-QRS-T axes 44, 75, 16
- QRS duration 100 ms
- QT/QTc 456/447 ms

Figure answer 4-9

Rate and rhythm?	Atrial fibrillation at 115 bpm
Pathologic Q waves?	III, aVF
ST-segment elevation?	II, III, aVF, V_5, V_6
ST-segment depression?	I, aVL, V_1–V_3
T-wave changes?	Inverted V_1, V_2
Voltage criteria for LVH?	No
QRS width?	104 ms
Reciprocal changes?	I, aVL
STEMI?	Yes
Interpretation:	STEMI, inferolateral. ST elevation noted in II, III, aVF, V_5, and V_6. ST depression in V_1–V_3 suggests possible posterior involvement, consider obtaining posterior leads. Obtain V_4R to assess for RVI. Does not meet voltage criteria for LVH. QRS duration within normal limits. Obvious reciprocal changes in I and aVL.

- PR interval None
- P-QRS-T axes 999, 57, 99
- QRS duration 104 ms
- QT/QTc 364/416 ms

Figure answer 4-10

Rate and rhythm?	Sinus rhythm at 75 bpm with left bundle branch block
Pathologic Q waves?	
ST-segment elevation?	V_1–V_3
ST-segment depression?	V_5–V_6
T-wave changes?	
Voltage criteria for LVH?	No
QRS width?	144 ms
Reciprocal changes?	
STEMI?	Possible STEMI (definite maybe)
Interpretation:	Possible STEMI/new-onset LBBB. Does not meet Sgarbossa criteria. As always, consider clinical presentation and use ST trending or serial ECGs.

- PR interval 130 ms
- P-QRS-T axes 13, −16, 58
- QRS duration 144 ms
- QT/QTc 406/453 ms

Illustration Credits

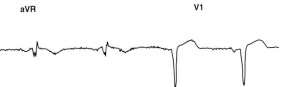

aVR   V1

FIGURE 1-2 Urden LD, Stacy KM, Lough ME: *Critical care nursing: diagnosis and management,* ed 6, St Louis, 2010, Mosby.

FIGURE 1-7 Methodist Hospital: *Basic electrocardiography: a modular approach,* St Louis, 1986, Mosby.

FIGURE 1-15 Butler HA, Caplin M, McCaully E, et al (editors): *Managing major diseases: cardiac disorders vol 2,* St. Louis, 1999, Mosby.

FIGURE 1-16 Patton KT, Thibodeau GA: /Anatomy and physiology, /ed 7, St. Louis, 2010, Mosby.

FIGURE 1-18 Modified from Urden LD, Stacy KM, Lough ME: *Critical care nursing: diagnosis and management,* ed 6, St Louis, 2010, Mosby.

FIGURE 3-2 Urden LD, Stacy KM, Lough ME: *Critical care nursing: diagnosis and management,* ed 6, St Louis, 2010, Mosby.

FIGURE 3-3 Lounsbury P: *Cardiac rhythm disorders,* ed 2, St Louis, 1992, Mosby.

Index